Dealing with an Alcoholic Parent

A Childs Guide to an Alcoholic Parent

Table of Contents

Dealing with an Alcoholic Parent 1

Introduction 3

Chapter 1: Understanding the Why 5

Chapter 2: Some Facts You Should Understand 7

Chapter 3: Risks Your Alcoholic Mother Might Pose 9

Chapter 4: Four Things to Remember 14

Chapter 5: Three Things to Avoid 17

Chapter 6: 11 Steps to Talk to Your Parent 19

Chapter 7: Some Questions You Might Have . 31

Conclusion 40

Introduction

I want to thank you and congratulate you for purchasing the book Dealing with an Alcoholic Parent.

This book contains proven steps and strategies that you as a child of an alcoholic parent can employ. It will guide you on how you can handle situations at home while your parent I probably drunk. Coping up with an alcoholic parent is not an easy task and you will have to make sure that you do not drain out of energy and motivation yourself.

You will need to create your own support system which you can fall back on when the need arises. This support system will be made up of safe people who will empathize and motivate you when the going gets tough. Safe people are those people in your life that you can trust and seek advice when you need to.

Here's an inescapable fact: children of alcoholic parent(s) are three to four times more prone to becoming an alcoholic themselves. But that does not mean that you will become an alcoholic too. The choice will always be yours to make. Whether you want to make the same mistakes your parents made or you want to learn from their mistakes and make a better life for yourself.

As you learn to handle and cope up with your alcoholic parent, you will so find different ways you will be able to handle stress and frustration that does not need alcohol. And this will help you handle stress as you grow up and make you stronger than the temptation to give in to alcohol.

Always remember, **you are who you want to be. Stronger than genetics, stronger than temptation and stronger than what people say.**

Chapter 1: Understanding the Why

You might be wondering why your parents need to drink so much. The common knowledge is that when a person is extremely sad, suffering from depression or just not able to handle stress, they tend to drink too much. It is more like a psychological thing. And you might feel sad or sorry for them. But then when it becomes a habit, it becomes a daily scene at home, you tend to become irritated or angry.

Understanding why a person drinks too much will help you understand your parents. It will give you further insight on how to handle them and even better, how to guide them to reduce and eventually quit drinking.

Here are a few points for you to understand alcoholism better and then you can relate as to which one applies to your parent(s):

- Research and studies show that alcoholism is a disease like any other disease. Alcoholism is not anyone's fault but a result of genetics, family history or a crucial life event.

- It can become a habit when the person is trying to cope with extreme situations like stress, money issues, emotional upheaval etc.

- Denial can be a big obstacle to quitting. If you are trying to make your parent(s) quit drinking and they happen to be in denial it will become very difficult. Denial is when they do not realize or do not want to accept that they have a drinking problem.

- Drinking might be a result of a stress or a temporary situation, but do not make the mistake of thinking that once the problem is over, once the stress is gone, the drinking will stop. No, it will not. It will become a habit.

Chapter 2: Some Facts You Should Understand

1. **It is a disease**: Alcoholism is a disease that alters a person's behavior when under the influence of alcohol. Additionally, the inability to control the amount of alcohol drunk makes it all the more difficult. That does not mean that you parent(s) is a bad person.

2. **Not alone**: You are not the only one who is having to handle alcoholic parents, there are many out there. So do not think that God has singled you out and punished you. Survey results show that nineteen million kids in US who are under 18 years of age live with alcoholic parents.

3. **Not your fault**: Resorting to alcohol is a personal choice and is their own inability to handle the situation. Their choice is not

because of you, but because of themselves. So never blame yourself for their drinking.

4. **Trust and talk**: When you have too many emotions, especially negative ones pent – up, you need to let it out or it will suffocate you. You will need a clear mind to handle your parents. So find someone you can trust and who is ready to listen to you. This person can be anyone – a teacher, a friend, your brother or sister, cousin, a doctor or anyone to trust enough to show your emotions.

Have you ever heard of Alateen groups? These groups are for kids. Here kids who live with alcoholic parents or relatives come together for meetings. They share their problems and give out suggestions to each other on how to make things a little better. They share their small successes or their hopes. This a great place for you to lighten your heart and pick up important tips that will help you too.

Chapter 3: Risks Your Alcoholic Mother Might Pose

Mothers are closer to a kid in the early years of his life. Not that fathers are not important, but since fathers stays outside the home for longer periods and most of a child's work is done by the mother there is a special bond created. A kid's expectation from his mother is also high. If the dad forgets the birthday he is ready to forget, but if the mom forgets to bake the chocolate cake it is not forgivable. The expectations are higher because the mother gives him unconditional love and care. That is how everyone sees their mother.

Now if you think of your alcoholic mother, things might become contradictory. How can a person who is supposed to love and care for you and also become a victim of alcoholism. And then you might feel frustrated and lonely because she isn't giving you the time and care you deserve.

The reality of alcoholism is that it doesn't differentiate their victims in terms of gender, age, race, nationality or any such groups and that is a sad reality you will have to accept.

Now that you have accepted it, you will also have to understand that there are certain risks that your mother poses and you will have to take ownership and take care of it.

Here are some of the dangers you need to know:

- Secret: Yes, you might be watching your mom drink at parties or at home when her friend come over. Gradually the drinking continues after the parties or after her friends have left. But you don't really see her out of control. Whether it is ego or just embarrassment that stops them from accepting that they are addicted, they keep hiding the fact that they cannot control their drinking habit. As a result, they tend to do all the normal chores some of which a person under the influence of alcohol should not be doing.

Vehicular accidents or fire accidents due drunk mothers are common news that makes the headlines frequently. If you realize that your mother has been drinking too much though she will not accept it, stop her from getting behind the wheels. Driving will be dangerous. Also, she might offer to make you a snack since you are hungry, decline the offer, or rather offer to make it yourself, being drunk and working in the kitchen can expose her and others in the house to fire disasters.

- Baby: You know that your mother is expecting and you still find her having a sip or two every time she thinks she is alone. She is doing serious harm to the unborn baby. This damage to the baby before it is born is called *fetal alcohol spectrum disorder (FASD)* and can be any kind of damage to baby – physical or mental disorder and a lot of times these damages are lifelong.

Statistics prove that 40,000 babies are born with FASD in the U.S every year. When the mother drinks, alcohol also reaches the bloodstream of the baby. Therefore the alcohol content of the baby and mother are at the same level.

This is a point where you cannot be of much help to her. Try to seek help from some other adults who could speak to her. You could let your father know that she has been drinking or a friend she is close to. Or your friend's mom or the safe people in your life who can help you.

- Attention: She is not giving you enough attention and this is hampering your thoughts. Don't let it. It is not your fault that she is drinking. She is just not able to cope up with a load of things and she is seeking alcohol to help her. You could try to use some techniques to keep reminding her of her duties. For example, keep reminding her that she needs to pack your lunch, or give you a shower, or iron your clothes or search for a book for you. Gradually she might start realizing that you are feeling neglected and she might have second thoughts about her drinking. This is not a guaranteed process. Just a way to get to her.

Chapter 4: Four Things to Remember

1. **Having Fun**: You are probably thinking and thinking and thinking so much that you have forgotten that you need to have fun and relax. Do not worry yourself sick. Yes, there is a problem at home, but that is not the end of the world. Worrying too much will cloud your mind and will help negative thoughts to take root. Have fun and you will see things in a more positive way and handling it will seem easier.

2. **Confused feelings**: Yes, it is normal to be having contradicting feelings. On one hand, you are furious with the addiction, on the other hand, you are struggling to accept your parents because you love them. Because your parents are not able to give you enough time, you tend to feel alone, yet you know the reason they are resorting to

alcohol and you cannot blame them. You might feel embarrassed because of their behavior in front of your friends or with your teachers, but you cannot help defending them to your friends or teachers. It is normal, so don't worry about it. Everyone tends to have more than one feeling. You will figure out how to handle it eventually!

3. **Safe people**: Talk about your issues with someone you trust – that is a safe person in your life, it is not a weakness, but a way to strengthen yourself to handle the situation. Like mentioned earlier, you need a clear mind to handle the situation and take the right steps. Talking to someone will lessen the feeling of being alone, you will derive positive energy from the person's support and this safe person might just be the right person to motivate you.

4. **Engage**: Loneliness or just the feeling of being alone can be a killing feeling and you do not necessarily need to keep it that way.

And because you are faced with a difficult situation does not mean you have to keep thinking about it 24hours a day, seven days a week. Free your brain of all worrying thoughts. But that will not happen if you sit idly. So join various activities that interests you. Things that you can take part in after school or on weekends when you have ample time. For example: sports – basketball, softball, cricket anything, or join the boy or girl scout, or some environmental club so you spend time with nature – the best healer!

Chapter 5: Three Things to Avoid

1. **Your mind** is a powerful tool and what you believe is very important in shaping out what actually will occur. The fact that your parents are alcoholic does not mean that you will be too. Remember that most aspects of alcoholism are psychological and what you believe will decide your course of action. If you decide never to fall a prey to alcohol, you can avoid alcoholism. That doesn't mean you have to abstain and never touch it. But you will be strong to have a glass or two and stop.

2. **Your safety** depends a lot on you. Remember that when your parent are under the influence of alcohol they might not to be able to make the right decision for you. So you will have to take ownership of yourself. If your parents want you to accompany

them to some party where you know they will be drinking, try to decline the offer. If they insist and you are not able to decline, make sure that after the party it is not your parents driving you back home. Get someone else to drop you home, maybe a trusted neighbor, friend's parents or your elder sister or brother.

3. **Your attempts** to help your parents is the best thing they can have from a son or daughter. Find help and help them in a structured way. Pouring out their drinking or just simply watering them down is not the solution. A lot of kids think that's a good way, but it isn't, it will not work that way. F they realize it, it might just serve to anger them. You don't have control over their drinking and finding the freedom from addiction is a process which has many steps you will have to employ.

Chapter 6: 11 Steps to Talk to Your Parent

Once you have realized that your parent is an alcoholic for whatever reasons, you have to find ways to cope. No, it isn't easy to handle, but it isn't impossible either. Understanding them will probably help you to cope with their behavior better. Additionally a few right steps you take might lead them to actually start thinking about quitting and they might actually be able to, you never know!

Step 1: Understanding them

Try to think about what are the problems they are facing that are bad enough to make them resort to drinking. When they are intoxicated, it is easy to just forget their problems or just put their responsibility on the next person. They find it easy to blame everything on the lack of control. It isn't right what they are doing, especially since the control depends a lot on the person. But you will have to exercise empathy. Put yourself in their shoes and understand the struggle they are going through. This understanding will not make them quit or prove them right; it will only help you cope up with their drinking better. Remember that you have to take ownership of your life and you can't let this hamper your life.

Step 2: Talking

Remember that whatever they are doing, they still love you. They may have resorted to alcohol but that does not hamper the bond a child has with his parents. So use this bond to reach out to their heart. It will not work any miracle but it will help you take a couple of steps towards progress.

Figure out a time when your parent is sober and you are in a good mood (not irritated but can maintain your patience). Sit them down to have a good talk. Tell them how you feel when they start drinking and what all goes wrong when they become overly drunk. Let them know what they are missing out on in your life. Let them know the risks that are there when they are drunk. This isn't only about them quitting, but also about your safety.

- Let them know what things are acceptable, and what is not. Do not dictate it to them but rather explain why they are not acceptable. Let them know that if they do not start taking positive actions, you will probably have to take a step of your own like talk to others and get help for them or leave to stay with someone else or anything you can think of that will start them thinking.

- Trying making them talking about their problems and share their reason for drinking with you. Don't be hurt if they refuse though, because it is difficult for them to accept their weakness to their kids and it will take time for them to talk to you. If on the other hand they do tell you the problems, reason with them that drinking is not helping them solve the problem but rather complicating things and creating other unwanted issues.

- Encourage them to try to reduce their drinking. Maybe drinking only as much as they can handle and then gradually reduce from there. There isn't any point trying to convince them to quit at one go, it will not work. They have to try in a gradual process and it will help. Also offer to get them information on groups or clubs who have others like them and they speak with each other and help each other take steps towards quitting.

Step 3: No Arguments

The way you set up the atmosphere and your approach in the conversation you have planned will go a long way to decide the success of your attempt. If you lose your temper or end of arguing when they are drunk, it will only create problems. They will probably clam up to avoid further arguments. They will probably not even remember the contents of the argument yet they will remember that you guys had an argument. Your whole point will be defeated.

Try explaining things and reasoning it with care. Do not let it sound like you are telling them what to do and what not to. They will feel you are being disrespectful. Let your concern show and let them understand that your words are coming from care and concern.

Step 4: Consistency

It will pay in the long run to be consistent with your words and actions. If you are going to put conditions or consequences if they continue drinking, then make sure you execute. Therefore, before putting the consequences in front of them, make sure you will be able to stick to it. This will make them think twice the next time they have a consequence in front of them. Also, when you are putting forward the consequence, make sure you make it polite. Let them know that because you are no more able to handle their drinking you have to take actions if they don't.

Step 5: It is not your fault

You are trying to make a difference and help them quit their drinking. If you keep thinking that you might be the reason to their alcoholism, you will not be able to think clearly because you are too busy blaming yourself and sinking in self doubt. You can never be the reason for their drinking. It was their choice to make – face the issue or drink yourself to oblivion.

Step 6: Journal

Pent up feelings can crowd your mind and turn into stress. Penning down your feelings can a be great way to vent out frustrations and arrange your thoughts. It will help you to figure out things better and understand the situation. It will simply help you to de – stress when your mind is overtaxed.

You can either write down your feelings in a journal or you could use an online journal if you do not want your parents to find it out. Remember that in order to help your parents your mind should be at its optimum health. If you keep worrying all the time and pent it up, there will come a time you will explode and it will not do anyone any good.

Step 7: Plan everything

Intoxication can make your parent incapable of remembering the responsibility. If you are going out with them, make sure you make plans how you will be returning back home, especially if you have to return in the night. You probably know that your parents will probably be drinking. Either make sure your other parent will not be drinking too, and can get you back home or talk to your older siblings or cousins to come pick you up. Or you might ask your uncle or aunt or anyone else who would help you out.

Never forget to have a backup plans and options to get you out of difficult situations. As mentioned earlier, having safe people in your life is very important. They are your support system, do maintain that adequately.

Step 8: Your mind

Living with an alcoholic parent is difficult at all times and it keeps worrying you as to what they will do next. But when you find yourself thinking too much and you can feel the stress building, take a step back. Worrying too much will not help the problem anyways, so divert your mind and find ways to step away from the problems for some time. Maybe you can just go out with a couple of your friends, or join some sports club where you play regularly, or have a hobby you can work on. This will help your mind escape from the problems and relax a bit. So when you are back home, you would be calmer and in a better situation to handle any issue.

Step 9: Do not follow their footsteps

Yes, your parent decided to use alcohol to run away from issues or handle stress when it got out of hand. And you have seen the consequences are hugely undesirable. Please learn from their mistakes and never take to drinking to handle your stress. Yes, sometimes the stress of an alcoholic parent might seem unmanageable, but their numerous ways you can relax and handle your stress.

Remind yourself how your parents are when they re drunk and use that as the motivation whenever you think that too can resort to drinking. Remember, stress is just an excuse, it is the choices you make, that defines you.

Step 10: Never tolerate abuse

There are many cases of alcoholics getting violent and abusive. Once it starts it is unlikely to stop. Never accept violence or abuse as part of being the child of an alcoholic. It will either continue or even getting worse. So plan it out carefully and move out of the house.

Once your parent starts to become violent:

- Check out emergency numbers you need to have in case things get out of hand. Add these numbers on the fast dial list on your mobile. Addtionally, keep a list of these numbers in your bag for easy access in case you are out and don't have your mobile for any reason.

- Start saving money and keep this well hidden, they shouldn't find out. Either ask your parents for small amounts of money when they are sober and put together all your pocket money so that when you leave, you will have something to depend on before you get your footing right.

- Make sure of whom you are going to go to one you step out of your house with your bags. Talk to a couple of possible people who will be ready to have you with them. Talk to your safe people to get ideas on how you will sustain.

- Guilt should not have any place in this whole plan and therefore do not hesitate to leave if you have everything planned properly. You do not deserve to be hurt, irrespective of who is hurting you. Even your parents do not have the rights to abuse you. If you have siblings who are also going through the same problems, gang up and plan so that you have each others back when you guys step out. You might think that you are being disloyal to your parents by leaving, but your safety is more important.

Step 11: Say it out

Talking to people you trust is the best way to deal with the situation. The fact that you have someone who will understand you and not judge you will give you confidence that will help you to deal with the situation better. Speak to them and let them know how severe the situation at home has become. Seek prior permission to stay over at their place for a night or two if things get out of control at home.

These people, maybe a teacher, you are close to, your friend or his parents, the counselor at your school, your sports coach or anyone for that matter. This is a kind of backup you are creating for emergencies.

Chapter 7: Some Questions You Might Have

Your mind might be full of questions and you might not find the answers to all of that immediately. Some only your parents can answer while some the safe person in your life can help you with while some generally frequent questions are answered here.

1. **What is Alcoholism?**

    Answer: It is a disease that compels a person to consume large quantities of alcohol such that it affects the physical and emotional state of the person. Alcoholism is an addiction that cannot be controlled by the person in question until he receives help.

2. **How does it start?**

    Answer: The reasons or causes of alcoholism are different for different people, but the common factors are similar.

A person will resort to drinking if he is under extreme stress or anxiety. Intoxication will help him forget the stress temporarily and shrink away from their responsibility. That isn't the solution to problems, but that short relief is what they are looking for. Gradually, when they continuously drink, they become dependent on the alcohol. Eventually, when the problem is solved, and the stress is gone, they find that they are not able to do with the alcohol and that's how it becomes a part of their daily life.

Also, for some, easy access to alcohol, like frequent parties where alcohol is served or regular outings with friends and having drinks or just a habit of casual drinking at home can gradually make them dependent on he alcohol and then it becomes next to impossible to stop.

3. **How does it feel?**

Answer: How a person feels when he is drunk depends a lot on how the body reacts to the alcohol. Excess alcohol affects the behavior and emotion of a person. A person might feel happy, free, sometimes silly or bold. Sometimes they might become angry, sad, violent indifferent. These are the emotional aspects. Additionally, when the alcohol consumption becomes too high, it causes nausea.

Physically, the motor skills are hampered, so walking, talking or even standing in one place becomes difficult not to say about any other tasks. Extreme consumption of alcohol might result in vomiting or a blackout. Black out is when the person cannot remember anything that happened in the short period of time he was out. Hangover happens the next morning after the night's drinking.

4. **How do I know?**

<u>Answer</u>: It is difficult to detect or identify alcoholism until it gets really serious. But there are a few things you might see to let you know that there might be alcohol issues.

- Drinking becomes a must everyday, whether there is a party or not. Looking for excuses to get a drink after the day's work.

- Making and breaking promises to you have been repeating for quite some time now. He keeps making commitments by doing this or that, but keeps forgetting or just say he does not have time.

- Missing out on responsibilities like attending the parent – teacher meeting, or forgetting to buy groceries or packing your lunch box or anything that she usually does.

- If he frequently mentions getting caught by the law for drinking and driving.

- Says he is drinking as a way to de-stress.

- Doesn't stop the drinking even when it is causing issues with your other parent.

- Your parent might feel irritated or tired and complain of headaches when sober. It means that alcohol is required for the normal functioning too.

5. **Why don't they seek medical help?**

   <u>Answer</u>: When do you go to a doctor? Only when you realize and agree that you are not well. Firstly, your parent does not realize that there is a problem with him. For him it is okay to just drink. Gradually, when he realizes that it is a problem with him that is turning him to alcohol every day, he will make excuses for drinking. He will not be ready to accept that alcohol is the problem. He would rather blame his friend or his boss or your other parent or the job or the house or sometimes even you or your siblings. Never take this to heart as he is

just looking for something else to blame so that he does not have to take the ownership of his problems.

6. **What is the cure**?

Answer: The cure is easy: stop the drinking. But that is something that is next to impossible for someone who has been addicted for some time now. But it is not impossible. Your parent will have to start by reducing the amount drunk gradually until he can spend a day or two without any drink. If he gets help, they will take him through a step by step process to help him withdraw from the grips of alcohol. There has been a lot of cases where a person recovered from addiction completely and now lives a happy life without alcohol.

Try talking to your parents and inspiring them to get help and begin reducing their drinking. Use their love for you to motivate them to eventually quit.

7. **How can family help**?

Answer: Family can act as a support, providing the motivation and confidence to work towards quitting but they cannot cure the person completely. For a complete quitting and effective result, the person needs the help of a trained person who can efficient guide your parent to take the right steps towards quitting. Your family can help to convince him to accept the help and inspire him towards recovery, provide him with emotional support.

8. **What are the statistics?**

   Answer: Statistic shows that there are approximately 11 million kids that are currently in the US who have at least one parent who is alcoholic and a scary 19million kids who are victims of alcohol abuse. There are a lot of kids that are in the same situation as you are, so never feel like you have been singled out and served this sentence.

9. **Why is it a secret?**

Answer: Alcohol addiction is a kind of a weakness and weaknesses are aspects of a person that he will not want to expose to everyone, even to his son or daughter. Accepting that he has an alcohol issue might result in others judging him and that is what he is afraid of. A person is defined by his choices and resorting to alcohol is not a good choice and he knows it.

Alcoholism, also has a social stigma which might lead to the loss of job, distaste from other family members and it will also result in them losing respect from their kids.

10. **Will I be an alcoholic when I grow up?**

Answer: Whether you become an alcoholic or not will largely depend on the choice you will be making when you grow. Some people forget what they have learnt and some learn from what they see. For a person like you who has seen all that happens when a person becomes addicted, how much he hurts the people around him, and how much he hurts himself should be a big enough lesson for you to stop yourself from becoming the same.

That does not mean that you will have to abstain from alcohol. It only means that you drink once in a while because of a party or a get to together, but never drink for a reason like relaxing or stress. Whenever you might feel like drinking too much, remind yourself of your own childhood and how your parent became when she was drunk and how you felt about it.

Conclusion

Thank you again for downloading this book!

I hope this book was able to help you to clarify a few of the major questions that would have been doing the rounds in your thoughts. Understanding alcoholism and why it happens will help you reduce any resentment you have against your parent.

You have to always remember that it is never your fault that your parent has decided to take to drinking. It is their inability to handle stress and burdened under too many responsibilities that drives them to seek alcohol to relax. That doesn't mean that they are bad people, it only mean they are not strong enough.

Finally, if you enjoyed this book, please take the time to share your thoughts and post a review on Amazon. It'd be greatly appreciated!

Thank you and good luck!

Made in the USA
Middletown, DE
21 November 2017